The Fitness Goal Triad

How to Successfully Reach Your Fitness Goals

By Stephanie Eissinger, MA, LCPC, CPC

This is a 1st edition.

The Fitness Goal Triad
How To Successfully Reach Your Fitness Goals

A Sagebrush Coaching & Counseling Services, PLLC Book

PUBLISHING HISTORY

Sagebrush Coaching & Counseling paperback December 2015

For Information Address: www.sagebrushcoaching.com

Table of Contents

Acknowledgments

This book is dedicated to my husband, Mark,
and my daughters, Rio and Nocona.
I can never thank them enough for their support and
encouragement.
Even on the days when I was doubting myself,
their faith in me never waivered.

INTRODUCTION

Embarking on a fitness journey is exciting and intimidating at the same time. The excitement comes when you visualize your life AFTER you've put in the time and effort to make healthy changes and what your future self looks and feels like. The intimidating part comes from visualizing the hard work itself, the sacrifices, and the requirement of getting out of your comfort zone that's necessary for true change to happen.

Plus, change is scary. Change implies "giving up" certain things that you're attached to. Getting "fit" means breaking old habits. It means eating differently, feeling and behaving differently, thinking differently, and looking at yourself differently. *Wow, that does sound intimidating!*

But it's possible to reframe how you view your fitness journey. Instead of seeing it as a grueling, deprivation filled obstacle course, you can mentally go to your "Spin Room" and put a positive *spin* on your view of the process. You can CHOOSE to look at it from a positive viewpoint that focuses on all the fabulous things you'll be gaining by getting fit.

Here are some examples of what you'll be gaining:

- new, healthier habits
- increased physical and mental strength
- increased emotional intelligence
- increased self confidence
- increased self esteem
- increased self respect
- increased self worth
- a healthier, toner body
- a healthier mindset
- a healthier emotional experience
- trust in yourself and your body

- a slowdown of the aging process
- better balance in your life
- improved mobility, endurance, and physical balance
- improved mental and physical flexibility
- a decrease in physical and mental stress
- an increase in physical and mental energy

I hope thinking about all the amazing benefits you have to gain from making the changes and doing the work required to find your optimal level of "fit" has *fired up* your motivation and commitment to taking care of yourself. It's the best investment that you'll ever make!

To get the most out of this book – set realistic goals for each of the 3 fitness components and put them into action. The successes you obtain in one area will support your efforts in the other two. Get an accountability partner to keep you honest and to celebrate your successes with. And, finally, believe in yourself...you have it within you to build a healthier, happier life.

Stephanie E.

CHAPTER ONE

The Fitness Goal Triad: Body, Mind & Emotional Fitness

"Start from the heart. The greatest journeys begin on the inside."

Eleanor Brownn

Traditionally, achieving fitness goals simply meant exercising our physical bodies to lose weight, gain muscle, and build endurance. This traditional definition doesn't take into consideration how thinking and emotions factor into the picture. By neglecting these two factors, the traditional approach too often leads to disappointment, shame and disenchantment with the body fitness process. People quickly get discouraged and give up. They give up their efforts to achieve a healthier, more physically fit body. They quit trying to meet healthy weight goals. And they lose the motivation to make other healthy lifestyle changes.

The Triadic Approach to reaching your fitness goals that I'm proposing takes all three factors into account: body fitness, mind fitness, and emotional fitness. Each of these fitness components influences and is influenced by the other two. This interconnection makes it extremely difficult to make permanent progress in one area without making improvements in the other two. Therefore, the quickest, most enduring way to find and maintain your fitness success is to address all three areas and how they interact.

Being fit means taking care of your mind and your body...exercising, nourishing and strengthening both. It also means increasing your emotional fitness.

Your emotional state and your mindset affect how you behave towards your body. How you treat your body affects your body fitness. If you're in a *good place* mentally and emotionally, you'll treat yourself and your body with the love and respect it deserves. You'll fuel your body with nutritious food. You'll strengthen it by exercising. You'll attend to physical health issues. And, you'll "talk" to yourself in a kind, accepting, and encouraging manner.

If you're in a bad place mentally and emotionally, you'll do just the opposite. You'll punish your body with "junk" food or starve it. You'll neglect it by not working out or addressing medical issues, allowing it to grow weak and physically deteriorate. And, your self-talk will be negative, judgmental, harsh, and self-critical.

Picture your thoughts, feelings and behavior making up the three different angles that define a triangle. If you change one angle, it changes the other two.

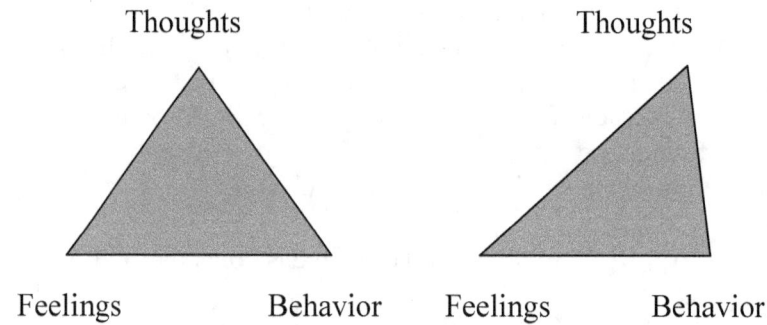

| Thoughts | Thoughts |
| Feelings | Behavior | Feelings | Behavior |

Examples of how this would look in the real world:

The following examples are all based on the same "triggering" event, but have very different outcomes. A triggering event is something that sets your thoughts racing off into either a positive or a negative spiral. It can be either internal (something inside you) or external (something that happens in your environment). If your mind fitness is operating at an optimal level, you're able to take the event in stride and manage your thoughts and the corresponding emotions, you can stay neutral and prevent your thoughts, feelings, and behavior from spiraling out of control.

Event: You gained two pounds since the last time you got on the scale.

Thoughts: "I'm such a fat cow. I'm a worthless loser that can't do anything right. What's the point of working out and trying to eat healthy? I gain weight just by looking at a food."

Feelings: You feel hopeless, ashamed, dejected and empty inside.

Behavior: You pull on baggy clothes and drag yourself to favorite chair with your computer and a container of chocolate chip cookies.

Same event: You gained two pounds since the last time you got on the scale.

Thoughts: "My trainer is such a liar, she said this fitness program would help me lose weight fast. I'm not losing weight, I'm gaining it! What a waste of time, energy and money. I'll show her..."

Feelings: You feel angry and resentful. Underneath your anger you feel anxiety, disappointment and fear.

Behavior: You skip your workout, order a large, greasy pizza loaded with extra sausage and pepperoni, and gorge yourself to misery.

Same event: You gained two pounds since the last time you got on the scale.

Thoughts: "How can I have gained weight? I worked out every day and ate healthy all week. I need to be perfect...I need to work out harder and longer and eat less. I HAVE to lose 10 more pounds before the party or people will think I'm a loser with no willpower."

Feelings: You feel anxiety, self-disgust, and fear.

Behavior: You skip breakfast and lunch, go for a run followed by a grueling workout, have a small lettuce salad with no dressing for dinner and then do some more exercises before showering and crawling into bed.

Still the same event: You gained two pounds since the last time you got on the scale.

Thoughts: "Dang, that was unexpected. But, the trainer did say that would happen once I started building muscle. And, I have to remember that it's normal for body weight to fluctuate a couple of pounds. I won't let this get me down or derail me. I'll just keep focusing on getting fit, working out and eating healthy."

Feelings: You feel discouraged and disappointed at first, but then determined, re-energized and hopeful.

Behavior: You go for a run before heading to the kitchen to whip up a nutritious meal and do a few counter push-ups and squats while you wait for your meal to finish cooking. You smile when you realize how many repetitions you can now do easily.

The first two examples show how negative thoughts and feelings can end in sabotaging your fitness and healthy eating efforts. The third shows how perfectionistic thinking creates negative feelings and the combination leads to self-punishment. The fourth example shows how nonjudgmental and realistic thinking promotes optimistic feelings and actions that are positive and healthy.

Body fitness includes aspects related to your physical health.

Body or physical fitness encompasses eating habits, exercise, and addressing any medical or physical issues that come up. Improving your body fitness initially requires:

- Exploring your relationship with food and your eating habits.

- Determining the type of exercise that fits your needs and that you'll enjoy (or at least, not detest!).

- Making adjustments related to any physical limitations, injury, or fitness level (one size does not fit all).

- Taking care of any medical issues (taking prescribed medications, going to doctor's appointments, and following the doctor's recommendations - modified fitness program, special dietary requirements, surgery, etc.).

- Evaluating sleep habits to determine if you're getting the appropriate amount of sleep.

The power of your thinking can not be underestimated...it either leads to success or self-defeat.

Mind fitness includes aspects related to your thought patterns, mindset and your mental health.

Mind or mental fitness refers to how your thinking processes and patterns affect your behavior and your emotional state. Increasing your mind fitness initially requires:

1. Self reflection to identify and explore your beliefs, values, self image, motivations, and habitual self talk.

2. Determining which thoughts and beliefs are self-defeating and/or self-destructive.

3. Self awareness of how your thoughts affect your mood and behavior.

4. Evaluating how your self image may sabotage your fitness goals. (e.g. If you see yourself as a couch potato or a loser you may subconsciously view your efforts as futile.)

5. Evaluating the accuracy of your body image. (Negative or distorted body images will undermine long term success.)

6. Examining your general mindset. (Are you optimistic or pessimistic? Are you positive or negative focused? How does your mindset interfere with or support goal attainment?)

7. Attending to any mental health issues you may be struggling with. (e.g. Depression, Eating Disorders, Anxiety, PTSD, etc.)

Emotional fitness includes aspects related to your feelings and your mood.

Emotional fitness refers to your emotional intelligence, your emotional state, how you feel about yourself (including your body) and your mood. Enhancing the level of your emotional fitness initially requires:

- Determining your emotional intelligence quotient.

- Identifying your feelings and how they affect your thoughts and behavior.

- Conducting an honest examination of how you feel about yourself and your body.

- Exploring how your thoughts & feelings work together to produce your mood.

- Examining how your mood affects your motivation level and your behavior.

Now that you're aware of the different aspects of each fitness component, it's important to have a quick discussion about how your general mindset, mood, and attitude can affect your motivation and the ultimate attainment of your fitness goals. I'll discuss those briefly in Chapter 2 before moving on to discuss specific goals for each fitness component in more depth in Chapters 3, 4, and 5.

This might be a good time to take a break, consider what you've learned so far, and do a few stretches!

Chapter 2

How Mindset, Mood, and Attitude Influence Fitness Goal Achievement

"If you're tired of starting over, stop giving up."

Anonymous

Your mindset is a belief about yourself and your most basic qualities. According to renowned Stanford University psychologist Carol Dweck, there are two basic types of mindset: a *fixed mind set or a growth mindset*. The first type creates a pessimistic attitude or frame of mind and questions about your adequacy while the second type creates optimism and motivation to gain knowledge, practice new skills and work on self improvement.

Someone who has a *fixed mindset* believes that their basic qualities, like talents and intelligence, are static or unchangeable. They don't believe that these qualities can be developed and think that talent will lead to success without any effort.

Someone who has a *growth mindset*, on the other hand, believes that through hard work and great dedication, these basic abilities can be improved upon. This type of mindset supports resiliency when faced with challenges and a love for learning. Operating from a growth mindset enhances motivation and productivity and will even make for better relationships.

Adopting a growth mindset means believing that *everyone*, no matter what their initial talents, aptitudes, interests, or temperament, can grow and change through training, experience and effort. Your true potential is unknown – who knows what you can accomplish with practice and hard work...."Look out, kettle ball, here you come!"

Having a growth mindset fosters your ability to crush your goals, to thrive under the most challenging of situations, and to add a facet of realistic optimism to your basic mindset. Your mind monitors your experiences, keeping a running account of what's happening to you, what it means and what you should do about it. Your mindset frames this information and guides how you interpret it. Simply put, it's the lens through which you filter and view your experiences.

If you have a fixed mindset, your internal dialogue is focused on judging yourself and others. If, however, you have a growth mindset, your internal dialogue is still sensitive to positive and negative input, but you are tuned in to how you can learn from it and what constructive actions you can take.

You may be saying "That's all great, but how do I change from a fixed mindset to a growth oriented one?" Carol Dweck suggests the following steps:

1. **Listen for your fixed mindset "voice."**

   ◆ When you approach a challenge, experience a setback, or face criticism – what is your inner voice saying to you?
   ◆ That voice may be judging your performance, talents, abilities.
   ◆ That voice may be telling you "I told you so. You were a fool for trying."
   ◆ That voice may be blaming others when you're confronted with constructive criticism.

2. **Acknowledge that you have a choice.**

   ◆ Realize that how you choose to interpret challenges, setbacks, and criticism is your choice to make.

3. **Respond to your fixed mindset voice with a growth mindset one.**

   ◆ Possible growth oriented responses:
     • "I may not be able to do it right now, but with practice I can learn."

- "Not trying is an automatic failure."
- "With passion and a whole lot of effort, I can get better at whatever I try."
- "If I don't take responsibility, I can't fix the situation.
- If I listen to the constructive criticism I can learn from it, even if it's painful."

4. **Engage in the actions inspired by your growth mindset voice.**

   ◆ Given time and practice listening to both voices, you can make the choice of which voice you decide to follow.
   ◆ The growth mindset voice will inspire you to:
     - enthusiastically take on your challenges
     - learn from your setbacks, get up, dust off, and try again
     - hear criticism with an ear for learning and the ability to choose whether or not you act on it

When you choose to develop a growth-oriented mindset, it opens your mind to the possibility of adding other positive facets to your basic mindset and attitude. It also increases your willingness and motivation to try new exercises, develop new healthier habits, and change your relationship with food.

"The tough part isn't getting your body in shape. The tough part is getting your mind in shape."

Unknown

A Mindset of Realistic Optimism

Realistic Optimism

One positive addition to your general mindset is "realistic optimism." If you cultivate a mindset that includes realistic optimism, you'll be able to keep making progress toward your goals, even if it's slow, and you'll look at obstacles and setbacks as challenges and opportunities for self-growth. Being a *realistic optimist* means being flexible in your thinking, focusing on the positive aspects of situations without ignoring the problems, and being solution-oriented.

It means planning for the worst, while hoping for the best. This mindset allows a wider perspective of situations and "outside the box" thinking. To be successful, you must believe that you'll succeed. To create and maintain motivation to reach your fitness goals, you need to be optimistic and believe in your ability to achieve what you've set out to do. The caveat is that you must be realistic in your expectations.

To generate a mindset of realistic optimism, you must evaluate different options, plan well, stay focused on your goals and objectives, utilize necessary resources, remain persistent, and take action to execute your plan to the best of your ability.

> **"I always like to look on the optimistic side of life, but I am realistic enough to know that life is a complex matter."**
>
> **Walt Disney**

Unrealistic Optimism

An *unrealistic optimist* holds the belief that success is a given and that no effort is required on their part for this to happen. They might even think the only thing they need to do is to radiate positivity and their goals will be reached. But, wishing doesn't make it so. My mother used to say, "If wishes were pennies, we'd all be rich." The same goes for getting healthier, *wishing* ourselves into "fitness" doesn't work worth a hoot! It takes specific goal-setting, consistency, hard work, and dedication.

"If you have a goal, write it down. If you do not write it down, you do not have a goal - you have a wish."

Steve Mariboli

Pessimism

Someone with a pessimistic mindset expects negative outcomes and anticipates that things will not work out for them. They believe anything good in life that comes their way will be far outweighed by the insurmountable obstacles and hardships they'll have to endure along the way. A *pessimist* is so consumed with focusing on the negatives that they generate a self-fulling prophecy of failure. They look for and expect the worst and by doing so, they sabotage their chances of success, no matter what their goal is.

A pessimistic mindset defeats you before you even get started. If you expect to fall short of reaching your fitness goals, your resulting behavior will make it come true. Your behavior will be influenced by the "*try factor*". Whenever my Coaching clients use the phrase "I'll try...," I immediately suggest that they change it to "I can..." or "I will..." to reinforce their commitment to completing the task. The slight change in wording takes the option of not completing the task off the table.

People often use the "try factor" in describing how hard someone works to accomplish something. The amount of effort you put into achieving your fitness goals is definitely a huge factor in whether or not you're successful. But, sometimes using the word "try" can also work against you.

The word "try" lets you off the hook and makes *not doing something* an option. Although it might seem like a minor distinction, it's important because it speaks to your level of commitment and determination to *get something done*, no matter how difficult it may be to accomplish. The language you use when you talk to yourself and to others about your fitness goals is a major determinant in how you think, feel, and act toward achieving those goals.

Examples of How Each Mindset Can Affect Fitness Goal Achievement

Realistic Optimist:
◆ goals are specific and realistic to the individual's time constraints, abilities, and current fitness status

◆ different options are evaluated in an effort to find the most effective one and to have alternatives if the first option chosen proves to be ineffective

◆ challenges and setbacks are expected and planned for

◆ focus is on achieving each step with the desired outcome in mind

◆ resources are accessed when needed

◆ goal attainment is pursued with excellence, persistence and daily re-commitment

◆ each success is celebrated, even the small ones

Likely Outcome:
- feelings of self confidence, self esteem, and self respect increase
- motivation to set and achieve new goals is renewed (even non-fitness related ones)
- high percentage of goal attainment

Unrealistic Optimist:
◆ goals are set too high and too vague (e.g. Lose 50 pounds – this is unrealistic for an initial goal and doesn't specify how it'll be achieved)

◆ inconsistent follow through and lack of progress made toward goal (e.g. Working out is "hit or miss" and little or no improvements are observed)

◆ challenges are unexpected and de-rail any forward progress or commitment

◆ needed resources aren't explored or accessed

◆ efforts are half-hearted at best; lack of determination or persistence

Likely Outcome:
- feelings of disappointment, disenchantment and discouragement
- continued lack of effort put into goal attainment; frequently changing goals or giving up on goals entirely
- low percentage of goal attainment

Pessimist:
◆ goals are set haphazardly, without any expectation that they'll be achieved

◆ each setback and challenge is viewed as a sign that goal attainment is impossible and they're used as an excuse for failure

◆ individual engages in behavior that's counterproductive to meeting goals (e.g. eating fast food several times a week – self-sabotage)

◆ unlikely to explore or access resources, if they're accessed, they become a scapegoat for lack of progress

◆ goals and the process of goal attainment become the enemy

Likely Outcome:
- feelings of anger, disgust, futility, and blame focused on external forces
- actions are undertaken with resentment and only if no obstacles are encountered, usually resulting in individual giving up
- very low percentage of goal attainment

"The pessimist complains about the wind; the optimist expects it to change; the realist adjusts the sails."

William Arthur Ward

Striving to develop and maintain a mindset of realistic optimism will not only help you attain your fitness related goals, it'll increase your chances of finding success in all areas of your life. Close your eyes and picture how productive you would be. Imagine striding confidently into the office and crushing your current challenges at work. Envision yourself calmly standing up for yourself in a difficult family or social situation. Picture running across the finish line of your first 5K. Can you feel the stress melting away?!

"Being in control of your life and having realistic expectations about your day-to-day challenges are the keys to stress management, which is perhaps the most important ingredient to living a happy, healthy and rewarding life."

Marilu Henner

Accomplishing goals not only reduces stress, it enhances your mood. The opposite is equally true. If you're able to improve the quality of your mood, it'll increase the chances that you'll succeed in meeting even your most challenging goals.

How Enhancing Your Mood Supports Your Body Fitness Goals

The combination of how you're thinking and feeling at any given time makes up your mood. If you're thinking about how big your thighs look in a pair of jeans and feeling hopeless about your physical appearance, your mood is likely to be depressed and withdrawn. You might snap at your significant other, reject their attempts to make pleasant conversation and retreat to the couch, remote and chip bag in hand.

But, if you're thinking about all the good things about your day, your mood is likely to be upbeat and outgoing. You might hum a little tune while smiling and moving energetically around the kitchen preparing a great tasting, nutritious meal. You might even take a brisk walk while dinner is cooking. Staying on track and accomplishing your daily fitness objectives further enhances your mood and your motivation to keep working to meet your overall fitness goals.

The simple truth:

It's easier to find the motivation and the energy to engage in healthy behaviors like exercising and fixing healthy meals if your mood is positive, "bright" and upbeat. It's much harder to find the desire or the mental and physical energy when your mood is negative, "gray" and depressed.

Your mood isn't etched in stone. If you're in a bad mood, do something about it.

Your mission - if your mood is negative, *do* something about it!

Your mood isn't etched in stone. Even if you've had a terrible day. You have the power to change your mood by changing the thoughts you choose to pay attention to. If you focus on positive thoughts long enough, how you feel will change too...Well, hello, good mood!

I'm ready to do something good for myself, how about you?

Enhancing Your Mood

You've had an awful day. It started off with you sleeping through your alarm and having to rush to get ready for work. In your haste to get out the door on time, you jerked clothes off their hangers and threw them on. This resulted in you feeling frumpy, disheveled and out of sorts all day. Your thoughts were centered on negativity and resentment of co-workers who looked and acted "put together" and confident.

On your way home at the end of your work day, you're feeling depressed, listless and totally unmotivated to workout or fix a healthy dinner. You experience an intense urge to swing thru a fast food drive in and binge watch your favorite television series while mindlessly scarfing a huge cheeseburger and fries. No doubt about it...you're in a crappy mood!

You can either give in to your urge to numb your emotions and engage in unhealthy behavior or you can choose to enhance your mood and re-ignite your motivation.

How To Give Yourself a "Mood Lift"

A "mood lift" is like getting a mastopexy to enhance your physical appearance, only it's an uplifting procedure for your mood. It has the added bonuses of being DIY (do it yourself), it can be done anytime, anywhere, and it's *a lot* less expensive than a plastic surgeon!

Ways to Enhance or "Lift" Your Mood:

1. **Take responsibility for changing it.**

   ◆ You have the ability to influence how you feel by choosing what you do.

   ◆ Choose to do something proactive and positive.

2. **Tune into your crappy mood and zero in on the driving force(s) behind it.**

   ◆ Sit down with the negative part of yourself and ask what it's upset about. Instead of fighting your feelings, figure out what it is that you need right now. (I'll bet it's not a cheeseburger, but it might be a good "sweat session!")

3. **Change your thinking.**

   ◆ Determine what you can and can't control.
   ◆ Accept the things you can't change and do something about the things you can.
   ◆ Identify what you've learned from the negative situation and figure out how you can use this knowledge in the future.

4. **Identify the positives.**

   ◆ Rather than holding on to the victim "story" that justifies your bad mood, re-write the story. Focus on positive aspects in the retelling. (You may even want to visualize closing the cover on the victim storybook and opening a new one in which you are the author. *Spoiler Alert*: This story has a positive, empowering ending!)
   ◆ Look for things to appreciate and be grateful for that may have gotten obscured by the unpleasantness of the situation.

Examples:

> The weather
> Friends and family
> Sympathetic co-workers
> Your health
> This book!

5. **Honor your natural temperament by engaging in activities that honor it.**

   ◆ If you're an introvert by nature – go for a solitary walk or run, curl up and read a good book, etc.
   ◆ If you're an extrovert by nature – seek a workout companion, ask your partner to help you fix dinner and chat about what was good about your day (avoid ruminating about the negative stuff).

6. **Practice perspective taking.**

   ◆ Seek to understand other people's point of view
     • Ask what they're feeling and thinking if you need clarification to help you see their side.
     • If you "can't" ask, for whatever reason – remind yourself that you're not the only one who has bad days and use your experience to build empathy.

7. **Listen to uplifting music.**

   ◆ Pick music that makes you feel like dancing or singing along.
   ◆ Avoid music that is dark or depressing.

8. **Use a motivational mantra.**

   ◆ Find or create a motivational mantra to provide a quick "lift" to your spirits (more on mantras in Chapter 8).
   ◆ Do this BEFORE you need it, don't wait until you're feeling too down to search for one!

9. **Change your body language.**

   ◆ Hold a smile for 60 seconds.
   ◆ Stand up straight, walk slowly with your head held high, relax your body but don't slump.

10. **Blow the stink off.** (rural Eastern Montana lingo – I'd wager it originated from Old Timers after a long winter of being cooped up in a cabin with no automated washing machines or hot showers available.)

◆ Get outside!
  • Feel the wind in your hair.
  • Smell the flowers.
  • Get a lungful of fresh air.
  • Appreciate the vastness and beauty that abounds in nature and that, in the scope of things, your day-to-day irritations and frustrations are downright insignificant in comparison.

11. **Read, listen to, or watch inspirational "stuff."**

◆ Videos, podcasts, audio tapes, etc.
◆ Self Help books or inspirational life stories

12. **Workout**

◆ Yep, there's no getting around it, working up a sweat by exercising elevates your endorphin levels and enhances your mood!

If all else fails, and you've tried changing your mood to increase your motivation level, you may need to bite the bullet and, as the Nike slogan suggests, Just Do It! Whatever "it" is. Taking action and getting something productive accomplished is empowering, satisfying, motivating, and mood enhancing.

As one of *my* Coaches frequently advised – "pick the thing you're dreading the most, but that you want or need to accomplish, and DO IT FIRST!" Everything else will pale by comparison.

On a personal note:

There are days when I'm so mentally exhausted and cranky that the last thing I want to do is workout or go for a run. On those days, I have to set my body in motion while keeping my mind focused on other things, climb the stairs to my exercise room and start lacing up my running shoes.

I don't allow myself to think about how tired I feel. I don't focus on how long I'm going to work out. I just go thru the motions because I know that it works...*every time*. Instead, I focus on how I'll feel when I'm done.

I also give myself permission to do an *easy* workout. I'll just walk or run at a very slow pace for a mile and see how my body feels then. Unless I'm in physical pain (the kind of pain when my body is screaming, "I need a break"), before I know it, I'm punching up the speed or I've decided to go out farther before turning around if I'm running outside.

I've never, *not even once*, regretted working out. I always feel better when I've finished a mentally or physically tough workout. (And I'm not a person who advocates using the terms "never" or "always.") I might still be tired, but it's a different kind of tired. Being physically tired after working hard is a pleasant kind of tired, not a mind numbing one. To me it's a *reward* for the amount of effort I invested in the activity.

There's something purifying about working up a healthy sweat. It cleanses the mind, body, and soul. It clears the mind of cobwebs and promotes effective problem solving and creative thinking. It's also a great way to release negative, toxic emotions. And, it relieves the tension we hold in our bodies.

The more I sweat, the better I *feel* physically, mentally, and emotionally.

A Matter of Attitude

If you think of confidence as a general attitude, developing skills in a broad range of areas in your life will boost your self-confidence in meeting your fitness goals. To increase your overall confidence level, you can deliberately engage in activities that require effort to achieve but aren't beyond your present abilities. Doing this on a regular basis will challenge the self-limiting beliefs you hold about yourself and the things you can and can't do.

Don't wait until you feel confident to begin your fitness challenge. Adopt a *growth mindset* that incorporates *realistic optimism.* Then take active steps to build *realistic confidence* and *self-efficacy* – the belief in your ability to achieve your goals.

Build realistic confidence in your ability to achieve your fitness goals by:

- breaking your overall goal into smaller, more manageable chunks or objectives (prevents you from feeling overwhelmed and gives you the opportunity to experience success sooner and more frequently)

- deliberately identifying goals that are difficult *and* possible for you to attain (builds sense of competence)

- engaging in activities that make you feel confident and competent (builds a feeling of mastery)

Taking doable steps toward smaller objectives (goal chunks) is one of the best ways to increase the optimism and confidence you have in your ability to reach your ultimate fitness goals. I'll discuss this in more detail in Chapter 6 "Guidelines For Setting Specific Goals."

Do You Need An Attitude Adjustment?

Mindset, mood, and attitude have been used interchangeably by some to describe a person's mental outlook. I believe they're related but not exactly the same thing. I've already talked about mindsets, mood, and cultivating a confident attitude. Now I want to take a closer look at other ways attitude plays into the picture of fitness goal attainment.

If you think of your attitude towards fitness as a stance, bias, belief, or philosophy it'll help you determine if your attitude has the potential to stand in your way. If your general attitude toward fitness is negative, chances are someone "gifted" you this book. If your general attitude on the topic is neutral you may have found this book at a resale shop for $.50 and decided "what the heck." But, if your attitude is positive and enthusiastic when it comes to the idea of fitness, you may have a stack of other fitness related books, a mound of workout tapes, and numerous fitness apps on your phone.

Taking the idea of attitude one step further, you can assess your stance on each fitness component discussed in this book (body fitness, mind fitness, and emotional fitness). Your beliefs about each component will influence the time and effort you spend on increasing your fitness level in that domain. If you believe, as I do, that they're interconnected and equally important to achieving life fitness, you'll expend equal amounts of time and effort setting and working on goals for each one.

Is Your Attitude One of Reluctance?

If, however, your attitude toward addressing mental and emotional health issues is one of avoidance or reluctance, you're probably going to balk at setting goals related to those components or you'll sabotage the ones that you do set. And, if you believe that there's no connection to how your mental and emotional functioning affect long term success in the area of physical fitness, your willingness to set and work toward goals will only extend to ones that fall squarely under body fitness.

To be really thorough, you can drill down even further and examine your attitude about specific areas that fall under each of the components (e.g. nutrition, importance of core beliefs, and mood enhancement). For instance, if your philosophy is that nutrition is important to overall fitness you'll be invested in fueling your body in a healthy manner and limiting your intake of "junk" food. (Notice I didn't use the word "eliminate" when referring to junk food – everyone deserves to have their favorite treat once in a while, in moderation, of course!)

To put the idea of *attitude adjustment* into practice, when you're at the point that you're contemplating your actual written goals, ask yourself:

- "What is my attitude, belief, bias or philosophy about this particular fitness area or goal?"

- "How might it benefit me to adjust my attitude related to this?"

- "How will not changing my attitude regarding this prevent me from obtaining lasting results on my other fitness goals?"

If you ultimately decide that you're in need of an attitude adjustment:

Adopt an attitude of experimentation. When you think in terms of "Let's see if I can..." your mind starts looking for solutions to your challenges. An experimental attitude opens you to new ideas, new approaches, and new ways of feeling. It gives you the mental room to change your mind....

I've included an Exercise Attitude Assessment starting on the next page to help you clarify what your current attitude toward physical exercise is so you can consciously work on changing it to support your fitness goals if necessary.

Assess Your Attitude About Physical Exercise

To get a clearer picture of your attitude toward physical exercise, complete the sentences below:

I exercise when...

I don't exercise when...

Exercise makes me feel (circle the ones that apply, add your own if needed):

strong	enthusiastic	fat	empowered
energized	old	thin	toned
muscle	sore	in control	powerful
healthy & fit	tired	young	disgusted

release from toxic stress and/or emotions

_____   _____   _____   _____

The last time I exercised was...

Afterward I felt...

I would exercise more, but...
(list all of the reasons you can think of that get in the way of you exercising)

I enjoy (physical activity)...

I would like to try (physical activity)...

Summarize how you think and feel about exercise:

Now you have a clearer picture of your exercise mindset and the challenges you face in achieving your physical fitness goals. This knowledge gives you the opportunity to proactively shift your mindset and figure out solutions to the obstacles (internal & external) that may get in your way.

Chapter 3

Body Fitness Goals

Healthy eating and living includes, not only eating nutritious foods that fuel your body, but engaging in activities that strengthen and tone your muscles, and attending to any medical or physical issues when they come up. To acquire your optimal body fitness, you need to feed your body with a variety of healthy foods and provide it with the physical exercise it needs to grow stronger and have more endurance.

Body Fitness

With the health and fitness craze and the media's emphasis on having the perfect body, it's easy to recognize and understand the physical fitness aspect of body fitness. Articles and advertising abound about the latest workout routine or video that promises to tone and shape and contort you into the "ideal" body shape. I'm not advocating for any of them...that's not to say that some of them don't deliver on their heavily marketed promises...rather, it's to say that each one of you has to discover the physical activities that you really like doing and that do what you want them to do.

Ask yourself what your true fitness goals are in relation to your physical body. Then use your answer to inform the activities you choose. Achieving overall fitness and health is best done by engaging in a variety of activities that include some cardio (at whatever level is appropriate for you), some targeted to increase flexibility, and some weight or resistance training. (My personal preference is body weight exercises like planks and lunges.)

A key ingredient to remaining motivated for the long term is to find ones that you love or at least don't mind doing.

Whether or not weight loss is a goal, a physical fitness regimen is generally more effective if you challenge your body by doing different routines or increasing the intensity or number of reps of your current routine as things become easy for you. If you're never out of breath or a little sore after a workout, you probably haven't challenged your body enough for your workouts to continue to be effective.

For example, my favorite form of physical exercise is running. To keep it challenging and decrease any chances I'll get "bored" or that running will cease being a stress reliever and will become a source of stress instead, I *loosely* follow this weekly routine:

> **SUNDAY:** Anaerobic exercises* before breakfast. Long, slow run followed by stretching. Recovery yoga before bed.

> **MONDAY:** Anaerobic exercises before breakfast. Short, recovery run and body weight exercises.

> **TUESDAY:** Anaerobic exercises before breakfast. 45-60 minute run.

> **WEDNESDAY:** Anaerobic exercises before breakfast. HIIT (High Intensity Interval Training) treadmill workout. Body weight exercises or Runner's Yoga routine.

> **THURSDAY:** Anaerobic exercises before breakfast. 45-60 minute outside hill run. Recovery Yoga before bed if I'm sore. (Where I live, every outside run is a "hill" run!)

> **FRIDAY:** Anaerobic exercises before breakfast. Whatever kind of run I feel like. Body weight exercises or Runner's Yoga routine.

> **SATURDAY:** Anaerobic exercises before breakfast. Day off of "formal" workout.

*Anaerobic exercises strengthen muscles by forcing them to work very hard for a brief time without using oxygen. They are a form of resistance training.

With my bent toward perfectionistic thinking and my competitive nature, I have to monitor myself to be sure that I'm not "upping the ante" too much and that I'm *listening* to my body.

I had to sit myself down for a good "talking to" recently. I needed to remind myself that, since I wasn't currently training for a half marathon, I didn't need to be logging 8 plus miles every day...that it was much better for my overall health to back off the mileage. Instead, I needed to increase the time I spend on body weight exercises and strengthening yoga. My body is still thanking me!

**This is NOT exercise advice, it's merely an example of how I've built movement (and stress management) into my life in a way that works for me.

The point is to make "moving" a part of your routine – make it a habit that enhances your quality of life.

Something that brings you pleasure, not anxiety and stress. What point is it to spend hours slaving and sweating through a workout regimen that makes you miserable – one that looms like a black cloud over your "to-do list" or takes over your life, becoming an obsession driven by something other than living a healthier life?

Physical movement is a key to optimal life functioning, but too often it becomes something to drudge through and dread.

I'm advocating for *weaving movement into your lifestyle in a way that energizes you and gives you a feeling of pride and accomplishment* from seeing positive changes in your health and muscle tone. Changes that give your self-confidence a boost and the knowledge that you're taking care of yourself.

No matter how "in shape" or "out of shape" you think you are, you can inspire yourself and others by taking the first steps on your journey to life fitness.

Body Fitness Areas to Target With Goals

To achieve body fitness you need to consider three broad categories to target:

1. Eating/Food
2. Exercise
3. Medical Issues/Physical Injury

Once you've defined broad goals that you want to attain, you need to break these into smaller specific goals or objectives to prevent yourself from being overwhelmed and to promote progress and build a foundation of success to enhance your confidence and help you stay motivated along your fitness journey.

As you're refining your body fitness goals and objectives, you'll want to consider these specific areas to target:

◆ **Your relationship with food and your eating habits**
- dietary and nutritional goals
- emotional and stress eating
- food as fuel rather than punishment, therapy or reward

◆ **Type, amount and frequency of exercise**
- cardio
- flexibility
- endurance
- strength

◆ **Medical, injury and/or physical therapy related (if applicable in your case)**
- this includes listening to your body and backing off when you need to and getting enough sleep and recovery time

- this also includes following Doctors' advice and taking prescribed medications as directed

When you reach your smaller goals and objectives, be sure to readjust them in order to keep making progress toward your larger goals.

Sample set of goals:

Eating/Food

1. Eat 2-3 servings of different fruits and 2-3 servings of different vegetables each day.
2. Explore the underlying cause of my emotional eating in biweekly sessions with a qualified Coach or Counselor.

Exercise

1. Run at least 3x per week for 30 minutes. (cardio and endurance)
2. Attend yoga classes 2x per week. (flexibility)
3. Do a body weight exercise routine 3x per week. (strength)

Medical/Injury

1. Progressive relaxation each night before bed to improve sleep and relieve stress.
2. Take medications as prescribed.

**Tips on how to set S.M.A.R.T. Goals are found in Chapter 6.

Chapter 4

Mind Fitness Goals

Next, let's spend a little time discussing mind fitness, or what I like to call having a "fit mentality" or fit mindset. Mind fitness refers to your habitual way of thinking, how you view the world around you, and how you talk to yourself. Your core beliefs and the life lessons you've learned color how you think, talk to yourself and what type of "lens" you see the world through.

Here are some questions to ponder that will give you a pretty good idea about how "fit" your mindset is and how well it's serving you in your quest for a healthier, happier life:

- Are you optimistic or pessimistic? Is your glass half full or half empty?

- Do you see the negative in everything? Or, do you look for the positive in even the gloomiest of situations?

- Is the world a bright, friendly place that's filled with opportunity? Or, is it dark and hostile, a minefield of hazards and people who are out to get you?

- When you "talk" to yourself are you loving and accepting? Or, are you harsh and critical? Be honest, is your inner voice your worst critic or your best friend?

- Do you have an accurate, healthy body image or is it negative and distorted?

- Do you have a healthy or unhealthy relationship with food?

- Do you have a positive, healthy mindset about food?

- What are your core beliefs about yourself, relationships, and the world around you? Do they fit with your values and your vision of who you want to be and the lifestyle you desire?

Self-reflection can sometimes be scary and painful, but the rewards far outweigh the discomfort, especially if making positive changes in your life is important to you. Whether your goal is to start a physical fitness program, alter disordered or unhealthy eating patterns, or learn to accept and love yourself and your body, it all begins and ends with how you think.

If your thinking is *"disordered,"* negatively focused and self-defeating, any changes or progress you make will be short-lived. Your habitual way of thinking will sabotage even the best of intentions. How you think is reflected in how you feel and in how you behave. To achieve long-lasting physical and emotional fitness you have to first achieve a fit mentality.

Happiness is yours if you start from the inside.

A "Fit Mentality"

You might be thinking, "That sounds all great and wonderful, but, what does a *fit mentality* actually look like?

Let me see if I can help paint you a portrait of someone who has achieved mind fitness:

- ◆ **Optimistic Realist:** This person hopes for the best but is prepared for the worst.

    - No doomsday gloom or rose colored glasses here!

◆ **Positively Focused:** Able to find the positive aspects of any situation and chooses to focus their attention there rather than on the negative aspects.

- For example: If this person was fired they would choose to see it as an opportunity to find a more satisfying job or further their education.

◆ **Positive, Accurate Body Image*:** Has an accurate perception of their body and has learned to accept, appreciate and love it.

- Regularly practices the Art of Self Love.

◆ **Healthy Personal Boundaries:** This person enforces personal boundaries that protect and respect themselves.

- Boundaries that protect their physical and emotional safety, their time, their self-respect, and their energy.
- Knows they're WORTH protecting!

◆ **Supportive Core Beliefs:** This person operates on a set of core beliefs that are aligned with their values and that support healthy life functioning.
- They've taken the time to review their core beliefs and have consciously determined which ones still fit for them and which ones they needed to discard or adjust.

  ➢ e.g. "I'm a beautiful person, inside and out." = KEEPER! vs. "I'm ugly and worthless." = DISCARD!

◆ **Has a Healthy Relationship with Food:** This person views food as fuel for their body, not as a means of rewarding or punishing it.

- Uses non-food techniques to self-soothe.
- Engages in healthy eating habits and patterns rather than disordered eating.

- Allows themselves food indulgences that aren't tied to emotions.
- Eats mindfully, aware of physical hunger and satiation cues.

◆ **Engages in Positive Self-Talk:** This person speaks to themselves in a positive, encouraging manner.

- Recognizes when their critical "inner voice" is tearing them down with negative self-talk and chooses to ignore it and listen to their positive inner voice instead.
- Able to use constructive criticism as a form of self love instead of as a self-destructive weapon.

Now that you know what a "fit mentality" looks like, you'll be able to recognize it when you see it in the mirror!

After taking the time for honest self-reflection:

- Are you content with your current mental fitness?

- Do you have a fit mentality?

If not, you've already taken the first step to changing that – self awareness gained from honest self reflection is a prerequisite to change. The second step is deciding what you'd like to change and prioritizing your "fitness" goals.

In order to change your life, you'll need to change your priorities.

Make sure your goals are specific, measurable, achievable, realistic, and time-measured; then evaluate and re-evaluate (S.M.A.R.T.E.R.). Start with one that you'll see quick results on and that supports all the others. After all, you want a success to feed your motivation!

Something else to ponder...your thinking has a direct affect on how you're feeling! More on this in Chapter 5: Emotional Fitness.

Mind Fitness Areas to Target With Goals:

To achieve mind fitness you need to consider three broad categories to target:

1. Thoughts and Beliefs
2. Body Image
3. Mental Health/Personality Traits

Remember that once you've determined broad goals, you need to break these into smaller specific goals or objectives that are manageable and will help you build confidence and mastery.

As you're refining your body fitness goals and objectives, you'll want to consider these specific areas to target:

◆ **Habitual thought patterns**

- Core beliefs (determine which are self-limiting or self-defeating)
- Values (prioritize)
- Quality of self-talk (positive or negative)

◆ **Motivations**

- Both surface motivations and underlying ones
- Long term and short term motivation

◆ **Mindset**

- Growth or fixed?
- Unrealistically optimistic, pessimistic or realistically optimistic?
- Attitude toward fitness in general and to each component separately (body, mind, & emotional)

◆ **Body Image**

- Positive or Negative?
- Accurate or Distorted?
- Healthy or Unhealthy?

◆ **Mental Health Issues**

- Are there mental health issues that need to be addressed? (Anxiety, Depression, Obsessive Compulsive, etc.)
- Are there personality traits that might work against you? (Perfectionism, Procrastination, etc.)

If you find that your list of smaller goals is, in and of itself, overwhelming, prioritize these objectives. First things first. Work on the goals that will set a solid foundation that supports your ability to achieve all the others. For instance, if you have a fixed mindset to begin with, you'll have a difficult time believing that you can improve on the assets you already have.

Sample set of goals:

Thoughts and Beliefs

1. Explore core beliefs and write down self-limiting and self-defeating ones by next Tuesday.
2. Write down top 10 values and put them in order of priority by next Tuesday.

3. Write down negative self talk and what to say to myself to counter it every night before bed.

Body Image

1. Take Body Image Quiz by tomorrow night.
2. Write down three things I can do to improve my body image to share next week with my Coach.

Mental Health Issues /Personality Traits

1. Consult with a Coach or Counselor about developing a well-rounded Stress Management plan within the next two weeks.
2. Find or develop a personal mantra to use when my perfectionistic tendencies start interfering with my progress by the end of the weekend.

Pat yourself on the back when you achieve even your smallest objectives and, then, before you lose momentum, develop a goal to build on that success.

*Tips on how to set S.M.A.R.T. Goals are found in Chapter 6.

Chapter 5

Emotional Fitness Goals

Being emotionally fit is just as vital to a healthy lifestyle and goal achievement as body and mind fitness is. The combination of how you're thinking (mindset) and feeling (emotional state) at any given time has a direct affect on your behavior. And, your behavior, in turn, either promotes or undermines your efforts to obtain body fitness.

Emotional fitness is a *state of being* that includes your ability to identify, appropriately manage, and learn from your emotions. It's being able to stay away from negative thinking and focus on being creative and constructive. Being emotionally fit also means having the ability to take control of your choices and having the inner strength to be who you want to be. These abilities stem from what David Goleman calls your "emotional intelligence."

How high your emotional intelligence quotient (EQ) is depends on how well you function in the following areas:

- **Self-Awareness:** your ability to recognize your emotions and the effect they have on others

- **Self-Regulation:** your ability to manage or control your emotions

- **Goal-Setting:** your ability to set clear goals

- **Positive Attitude:** your ability to maintain a positive attitude

- **Perspective:** your ability to see things from another person's point of view, as well as your own

- **Social Skills:** your ability to understand, empathize, and communicate well with others

- **Stress Management:** your ability to deal with stress in a healthy manner

- **Motivation:** your ability to defer immediate gratification in order to achieve long term goals

It makes sense that the higher your EQ is, the higher your overall emotional fitness level will be. And, the higher your emotional fitness level is, the less likely you'll be to engage in emotional eating and other behaviors that sabotage your fitness goals. People with a high EQ have a positive attitude, are able to motivate themselves, manage their emotions well and rarely fall into negative, self-defeating thought patterns (disordered thinking).

Individuals with a low EQ often find themselves being "emotionally hi-jacked" by their intense feelings. When strong emotions seize control, individuals are unable to access rational thoughts and are likely to overreact to situations, creating further stress and negative outcomes.

Learning more about yourself through self-reflection and self-awareness gives you information on how your habitual way of thinking affects how you feel about yourself and your body. And well developed emotional management skills allow you to deal effectively with strong emotions so they don't interfere with you ability to achieve your fitness goals or live a healthier life.

In middle school and high school, my emotional intelligence quotient was fairly low in some areas. I'd learned not to show or talk about my emotions or problems and to put a "mask" on. I'd learned that being emotional and vulnerable was unacceptable. I knew how to "manage" my strong emotions externally, but not how to deal with them internally. As a consequence, I was engaging in self-destructive behaviors.

It wasn't until I was entrenched in disordered eating behavior, that included severely restricting my food intake, and a disordered thinking pattern that included thinking I was responsible for everyone else's happiness, that I was forced to take a good look at myself and my part in my misery.

I was sitting on the floor of my bathroom with a handful of pills thinking that no matter what I did, it was never good enough. I didn't really want to die...but I was so exhausted from carrying the heavy burden of trying to be perfect that I knew I couldn't keep doing what I was doing. I had a choice to make – either figure out what to do differently, or, go ahead and swallow the pills.

I could hear people moving around in the house, going about their routines, all of them assuming that I was doing what I "should" be doing (homework, chores, etc.). I realized at that moment just how alone I felt. How lonely and depressed and worthless I'd been feeling for a long time. And, that no one had any idea that I was in crisis.

The noise of the "outside" world went away and I was left facing myself and that handful of pills. I finally understood that I'd been slowly destroying myself to gain the approval of others. I started thinking about all the things I was really great at and all the things I was grateful for. And, an amazing thing happened – I GOT ANGRY!

I got angry at my family, my friends, and my boyfriend for not appreciating me for who I was, as I was. *I got even angrier at myself for doing the very same thing!* How could I expect others to appreciate and love me when I didn't appreciate and love myself?

I remember my next thoughts very clearly. I remember thinking "The hell with them, I'm going to stick around and show them just how great I am, with or without their support and approval." (Quite a statement from a "perfect" young woman who didn't typically use swear words.)

Your emotional pain can twist you...turn your pain into wisdom instead.

I decided: I'd start listening to, respecting and learning from my emotions. I'd take care of and protect myself. I'd be successful on my terms. I'd be proud of my accomplishments. And, I'd be true to who I was deep down inside. I'd be my best self – for myself!

My EQ increased several points that day!

Allowing myself to accept, feel and learn from my anger, gave me with the motivation I needed to flush the pills down the toilet and to start making desperately needed changes to my thinking and my behavior. Don't get me wrong...the changes took time and I still struggle with disordered eating and thinking when life gets tough, but with continued self awareness and regular self-reflection I'm able to deal with them proactively.

Don't wait until you've hit rock bottom like I did, today is a GREAT day to start improving your Emotional Fitness and increasing your EQ score!

Emotional Fitness Areas to Target With Goals:

To achieve emotional fitness you need to consider three broad categories to target:

1. Emotional Intelligence
2. Feeling, Thoughts, and Behavior Connection
3. Mood

Identify any deficits in your emotional fitness and then develop specific goals to strengthen these areas. Managing your emotional state and learning how to influence it positively will help you continue working toward your goals even on difficult days when you're struggling to feel motivated.

As you're refining your emotional fitness goals and objectives, you'll want to consider these specific areas to target:

◆ **Increasing your Emotional Intelligence Quotient**

- Ability to identify, express and manage strong emotions
- Ability to see another's point of view and empathize with their feelings
- Social Skills
- Stress Management
- Ability to stay motivated to work toward goals
- Ability to maintain a positive attitude

◆ **Connection between feelings, thoughts and behavior**

- How what you're feeling helps or hinders your progress
- How your feelings affect your ability to maintain motivation
- How your feelings can lead to self-defeating behaviors

◆ **Mood**

- How your thoughts and feelings interact to influence your mood
- Developing ways that you can enhance your mood
- Are you prone to depressed or "bad" moods?
- Do your moods interfere with your motivation level?

Sample set of goals:

Emotional Intelligence

1. Fill out feelings section of Thoughts, Feelings & Behavior Log for 7 days.

   - Pay attention to feelings (primary, secondary and tertiary)* as they come up
   - Put feelings down in Thoughts, Feelings, & Behavior Log
   - Write down what was happening at the time
   - After 7 days, add thoughts and behavior to Log.

*Primary feelings are the most easily identified (e.g. Anger, sadness, fear). Secondary and tertiary feelings are often "masked" by primary feelings (e.g. Rejection, embarrassment, hurt) They may be harder to pinpoint and include an element of vulnerability.

2. Choose 2 different stress management techniques and use daily for 2 weeks.

   - Write down how I felt before and after using each technique to determine effectiveness.
   - Evaluate effectiveness.

Feelings, Thoughts and Behavior Connection

1. Add thoughts and behaviors to Thoughts, Feelings & Behavior Log. Fill Log out completely for 14 days. (After filling out feelings section for 7 days)

Mood

1. Give myself a "mood lift" each time I recognize that I'm in a bad mood, documenting the mood enhancing action taken and how well it worked on a 1-10 scale (1 = Not at all effective; 10 = Very Effective)

2. If I'm unable to change my mood, I'll do what I need to do anyway, documenting how I feel before and after I'm finished.

At this point you're probably anxious to sit down and write out your fitness goals (if you haven't already), but, I want to share a little more information with you first. It pertains to the *language* you use when formulating your written goals. Using the right language in written goals makes it easier to gauge your progress, identify and problem-solve obstacles to successful completion, and builds in accountability. The next chapter outlines the specifics on how to write effective goals using the acronym S.M.A.R.T. as a guide.

Are you ready to set your life fitness goals???

Chapter 6

Guidelines To Setting Specific Goals

"Goals are dreams with deadlines."

Anonymous

Now that you've explored each fitness component in detail and have pinpointed the specific things you need and want to address in each one, you're ready to develop your fitness plan that incorporates all three components. You're ready to set realistic goals, renew your commitment to yourself, and take action.

If you want to make changes, get healthier, and grow as a person, you have to set goals. Otherwise, you're just allowing life to happen and any changes that occur will be orchestrated by someone or something outside of yourself. You can't complain about how things are for you if you're unwilling to take responsibility for yourself or the necessary action steps for making the changes *you* want.

One of the things that makes goal-setting more successful is focusing on what you're gaining by making the changes instead of on what you think you're losing.

"One reason people resist change is because they focus on what they have to give up, instead of what they have to gain."

Unknown

Without well defined goals and the determination to consistently do the work involved in reaching them, it's easy to get side tracked by everyday distractions. The next thing you know, you're a another year older and still out of shape. All those dreams about having a fit, healthy body that you love are still floating around in your head but are no closer to being reality.

"Almost every successful person begins with two beliefs: the future can be better than the present, and I have the power to make it so."

Anonymous

Developing goals and creating action steps gives you the power to make your dreams a reality. A goal is simply the outcome of a series of actions that are performed within a specific amount of time. If your goal is to walk on the treadmill for 20 minutes each day, then the actions to reach this goal are *making the time and performing the exercise every day.*

The goal is the end result you're hoping to achieve. The action steps are the vehicle that drives forward progress toward that end result. Specific action steps keep you focused and on track. They're also a means of monitoring your goal status and an opportunity to celebrate smaller successes that increase motivation, self-esteem, and self-confidence.

"A goal without a plan is only a wish."

Anonymous

Creating a Goal Plan

Creating an effective goal plan requires the inclusion of three elements:

1. well thought-out goal(s) that reflect your priorities
2. an action plan that includes smaller objectives (goal chunks)
3. a clear system for monitoring progress and accountability

Goals

When determining your goal(s) for each of the three fitness components, ask yourself the following questions for each area:

- ✓ What habits do I want to change?
- ✓ What aspects of my fitness do I want to improve?
- ✓ What do I want to learn?
- ✓ What are the most important things to do first?

The Language of Great Goals

Clarifying your goals is the first step to developing a great goal plan, writing them down in the most effective language is the second. Once you've clearly determined your goals and their priority (you can't do everything at once), write them down using the following language guidelines.

Guidelines for Effective Goal Language

To write an effective goal it should be positively focused, specific, measurable, and time framed. The following examples show you how to start with a basic goal and refine it to make it precise and effective.

1. **Even if your goal is to lose a negative behavior or habit, put a *positive* spin on it.**

- I will quit eating junk food. (negative focused)
  - ➤ I will eat healthy meals and healthy snacks. (positive focused)

- I will stop feeding my emotions. (negative focused)
  - ➤ I will learn 3 non-food ways to deal with my uncomfortable emotions. (positive focused)

- I will stop being a couch potato. (negative focused)
  - ➤ I will workout. (positive focused)

2. **Make the goal specific and measurable to enable progress to be monitored**.

- I will eat healthy meals and healthy snacks.
  - ➤ I will eat 3 healthy meals and 2 healthy snacks. (specific and measurable)

- I will learn non-food ways to deal with my uncomfortable emotions.
  - ➤ I will learn 3 non-food ways to deal with my uncomfortable emotions. (specific and measurable)

- I will workout.
  - ➤ I will walk/run for 30 minutes at least 3 times per week.

3. **Add a time frame.**

- I will eat 3 healthy meals and 2 healthy snacks.
  - ➤ I will eat 3 healthy meals and 2 healthy snacks every day. (time framed into 24 hour periods)
- I will learn 3 non-food ways to deal with my uncomfortable emotions.
  - ➤ I will learn 3 non-food ways to deal with my uncomfortable emotions by Friday of this week.
- I will walk/run for 30 minutes at least 3 times per week.

> I will walk/run for 30 minutes at least 3 times per week for the next two weeks, then I will evaluate if I need to increase the difficulty of this goal. (time framed)

4. **Be sure that your goal is achievable.**

   - Do I have enough time to work on this goal?

   - Do I have the necessary skills, strengths, abilities or resources?

   - Is my responsibility for achieving this goal stated in the written goal?

5. **Be sure that your goal is believable and realistic.**

   - Do I believe I can achieve this goal?

   - Given my knowledge of myself, is this goal realistic for me?

Goals need to be difficult enough to challenge you but achievable and realistic given your current circumstances. Taking the time and effort to set fitness goals that are individualized to you and the uniqueness of your situation may seem tedious, but I assure you, the results will be worth the effort!

When it comes to fitness goals, one size DOES NOT FIT ALL!

Poorly defined and written goals can lead to:

- boredom because they're too easy
- lack of progress because they're not specific or measurable or time framed
- frustration because they're unachievable or unrealistic

All three of these result in individuals giving up on their goals and returning to pre-goal behaviors. Once this happens, it undermines the person's self-esteem and self-confidence, making it less likely that they will try again or succeed in reaching goals in other areas of their life. Their fear of failure is reinforced and they go back to coasting and allowing life to happen.

Don't let this negative cycle happen to you! You can increase your chances of reaching your fitness goals by using effective goal language and double checking that the previous guidelines are met before embarking on your journey toward improved life fitness.

Goal Review

One easy way to initially review your goals for their potential to be effective is to use the S.M.A.R.T. acronym to assess it.

- S = Is this goal specific?

- M = Is this goal measurable?

- A = Is this goal achievable?

- R = Is this goal realistic?

- T = Is this goal time framed?

If your goal passed this initial S.M.A.R.T. test, move on to the next level of review. This is the part that I like to call the *Self-Reality Check*. It consists of three questions that require honest self-reflection and examination.

- ◆ Do I want to do it?
  - It needs to be something that you choose to do out of want, not because you "should" or because you're required to.

◆ Does it fit into my personal value system?
  - It needs to be important to you and aligned with your values.

◆ Am I motivated to achieve this goal?
  - Assess your motivational level
  - Ask yourself: Are there conflicting motivations that might sabotage my ability to achieve this goal?

If you answered "yes" to all three questions you are GOOD TO GO! If you answered "no" to even one of them, further exploration may be necessary to determine if the goal is worth setting.

"If it is important to you, you will find a way. If not, you will find an excuse."

Anonymous

Writing awesome goals is a skill you can learn that virtually guarantees you success, especially if they're part of an organized goal plan that includes a detailed action plan, a clear monitoring system, an accountability partner, and a game plan for dealing with obstacles and times of low motivation.

Action Plan

An action plan organizes your overall goals and breaks them down into manageable "goal chunks" or objectives. Succeeding at smaller goals that build on each other is one of the secrets of long term goal success. For example, if your long term goal is to lose 15 pounds (and this is an appropriate goal for you), then breaking this bigger goal down into smaller goals and setting specific objectives will provide you with stepping stones on your path to reaching that goal.

Example

Goal: I will lose 15 pounds over the next 6 months.

Goal Chunk: I will lose 3 pounds in the next 3 weeks. (Once this smaller goal has been reached you get to celebrate and then set a new one!)

Objectives:
1. I will walk for 30 minutes every night after work.
2. I will eat 3 nutritious meals per day.
3. I will do body weight exercises for 15 minutes each morning.

Think of the goal as the outcome you desire, the goal chunks as the baby goals that you need to accomplish first, and the objectives as the actions you will take to meet each goal chunk.

The cool part of action plans is that they are a "work in progress," not set in concrete. You can adjust the objectives if they're not working and you can move on to the next level goal chunk without having to change the goal itself. And, you get to celebrate and build on your strengths and successes all along your journey to reaching your bigger goals.

"Success is the sum of small efforts, repeated day in and day out."

Anonymous

Clear Monitoring System

Monitoring your progress and holding yourself accountable are important pieces of goal attainment.

Some goals are easier to monitor than others. It is easy to monitor whether or not you are walking 3 times per week, not so easy to determine if you are continuing to use food to numb your feelings. Here are some suggestions on how to monitor progress that can be tailored to meet your specific needs. Pick the system or method that works best for each of your particular goals.

- *Food Diary (that can include feelings before and after eating, triggers, percentage of healthy food vs. junk foods (80-20%) etc., depending on the specifics of the goal being targeted)

- *Thoughts, Feelings, and Behavior Log

- Track the number of days you go without engaging in a negative behavior

- Track the number of days or amount of time spend engaging in a positive behavior

- *Exercise/Running Log

- Journal about each time you felt the urge to eat when you weren't physically hungry, but decided to do something else instead

Ask yourself "If 10 unbiased observers were asked whether or not I reached the goal, in the way I've defined it, could they clearly agree?" If the answer is "YES," you've got yourself a measurable goal and a clear monitoring system!

Accountability

Following up with an accountability partner, such as a exercise buddy, supportive friend, Coach or Counselor provides you with extra incentive to work consistently on the action steps (objectives) of your goal plan. An accountability partner can help you review your action plan regularly, present alternative suggestions, brainstorm obstacles, increase your motivation, and celebrate your successes with you.

When deciding on an accountability partner there are a couple of things to keep in mind: 1) buddies and friends may go "soft" on you and let you off the hook, or even sabotage your progress out of their own insecurities, and 2) a Coach or a Counselor provides unconditional positive regard *and* accountability, is objective, knowledgeable, and invested in your success.

If you know yourself well enough and are honest enough to say "I need a lot of firm support, and, maybe even a little tough love, to keep me on track and to stay motivated" you may want to consider a formal accountability partner. If the cost of Coaching or Counseling is holding you back, think about what it's costing you to NOT change, to not reach your goals. When viewed in that light, the expense of Coaching or Counseling services is really a small investment. And the best investment you'll ever make is in yourself.

*You'll find a sample Food Diary; Thoughts, Feelings & Behavior Log; Exercise/Running Log; and Life Fitness Goal Plan in the appendix at the back of this book.

"Discipline is the bridge between your fitness goals and fitness success."

Felicity Luckey

Overcoming Obstacles

No matter how well thought-out and well-written your goals and goal plan are, you will encounter obstacles. They might be internal obstacles like self-doubt, disbelief, conflicting motivations, or fear of failure. They might also come in external form like limited time or resources, family conflict, chaos or crises. It's not a matter of if they'll crop up, but a matter of when and how you choose to deal with them.

You can use obstacles as an excuse to put your goals on hold or use them as a challenge that provides you with a chance for self-growth. A chance to brainstorm and problem-solve. Obstacles present a moment of truth. They force you to answer the question: How strong is my commitment level to meeting this goal?

Will you redouble your efforts, use "out of the box" thinking, and come up with a positive solution?

Or, will you retreat, blaming the obstacle for your defeat?

An Obstacle Crushing Mindset

Coming head-to-head with an obstacle is another opportunity to tweak your mindset. If you expect obstacles to be a part of the process of goal attainment, you'll be able to prepare for them rather than being caught off guard and easily discouraged. If you view obstacles as challenges or problems to be solved rather than insurmountable road blocks, you will meet them with creative thinking, an open mind, and a willingness to go the extra mile. You'll figure out how to go around, get over, or break thru them. The point being...you won't give up!

"I am stronger than this challenge and this challenge is making me stronger."

perfection-is-overrated

Chapter 7

The Motivation Misbelief

"Don't be upset by the results you didn't get with the work you didn't do."

Anonymous

A lot of people hold the mistaken belief that motivation is necessary for goal achievement. In reality, there are a lot of times when the only way to *generate motivation* is by taking action.

Motivation Misbelief:

- Action requires motivation.

Feeling motivated is nice and can make taking action feel less difficult, but it's not a prerequisite to taking action. Thank goodness or the dishes and the laundry might never get done! In reality, motivation is mercurial and fleeting. Especially the jump up and spring into immediate and enthusiastic action kind of motivation that comes from inside, not from external sources like a sink overflowing with dishes or not having any clean clothes left to wear.

The proof: Even if you don't want to do the dishes or the laundry, most of you do them anyway, and, before you're left with no other options. (My husband used to only use paper plates before we were married – his way of circumventing the whole motivation to wash dishes dilemma. He was so motivated to not have to do the dishes but have the kitchen clean when I got there, that he decided to buy his way out of it!)

For instance:

You watch an inspirational youtube video during your morning coffee break and you're all jacked up about starting a new fitness routine, easily passing up the lure of fresh bakery goods sitting on the counter. Then life intervenes. Your boss calls you into her office to "request" that you finish a time consuming work project before you go home that day. You're instantly deflated, defeated and unmotivated. Your plans for hitting the gym after work derailed. You think, "I might as well grab a doughnut from the break room on my way back to my tiny, depressing cubicle."

Even though your feelings of motivation dissolved with your increased workload, it doesn't mean you can't still take action. It just means that you'll have to make the decision to put on your workout clothes when you get home and exercise anyway. Even if you're not *feeling* it!

Even if you're tired, even if you feel like it's the very last thing on earth you want to do. TRUST ME...when you've worked up a good sweat, you'll be energized, in a better mood, and feel the *motivation* that comes with knowing you did something great for yourself.

If you wait to feel motivated before you work on your fitness related goals for the day, chances are you'll never get started, much less finished. Wanting to feel inspired before you act on your fitness goals can mean you'll still be waiting for inspiration to "arrive" a week, month, or even a year from now. To make changes in your life, you can't wait for motivation, you must take deliberate action, over and over again. Sometimes, the motivation comes once the action begins.

"If it's important to you, you'll find a way. If it's not, you'll find an excuse."

Unknown

If you find yourself consistently undermining or sabotaging your fitness goals, you need to ask yourself "What's the *true* or underlying motivation behind my actions?" "How am I being rewarded for NOT taking the actions I need to in order to reach my goals?".

- Am I only going through the motions to get my family and my doctor off my back or because I feel like it's expected? (true motivation)

- Does my significant other reward me with unprecedented attention when I eat junk food because they're afraid I won't want to be with them if I get in shape or because they don't want to make changes themselves? (rewarded with previously absent attention)

- Does my mother sabotage my fitness efforts because she doesn't want me to be more social and active and spend less time with her..showering me with fattening baked goodies and love when I visit? (rewarded by love, motivated by guilt to overeat unhealthy food)

- Does fear of failing motivate me to self-sabotage my fitness efforts? (motivated not to try out of fear of failure)

In the case of my husband and dishes, his true motivation was to get out of doing them, but have the kitchen clean when I came over, not to have a tidy house or a sense of order or feelings of accomplishment. The truth of the matter is, sometimes your efforts may be being influenced by unidentified motivations that are deeper or stronger than the desire you have to get fit. You may need to spend some time self-reflecting and dig a little deeper to determine if you're truly ready to transform your life.

Motivational Truths:

- You don't have to feel motivated to take action.

- Taking action leads to taking more action.

- Feeling consistently motivated to reach your goals would be fantastic, but it isn't necessary.

- Identifying underlying opposing motivations, including how your self-sabotaging behavior is being rewarded, is a key component to succeeding at any stated goal.

Your motivational level will ebb and flow. That's normal and to be expected. Enjoy and take advantage of the times when your motivational level is at it's peak, but don't let the inevitable motivational valleys stop you from making progress!

Chapter 8

Motivational Mantras

"The body achieves what the mind believes."

Anonymous

Your mind can be a powerful force for making you stronger, more determined, and more resilient...or it can be your biggest enemy, undermining your confidence and highlighting your weaknesses. You have the ability to decide which role your mind will serve. Will you decide to shape your mind into an even stronger ally...or will you choose to feed it with negativity, allowing the enemy to take root and grow?

Mantras are widely acknowledged to be an effective tool in training your mind to be your ally. A mantra is a motto, slogan or statement that's used as a guiding principle. You can use it to inspire you, to help you focus, and to motivate you when your struggling. Mantras can be used in business, athletic, fitness and/or personal settings.

Russell Wilson is known for using the mantra *"Why not us?"* in the pursuit of his goals as a leader and quarterback for the Seattle Seahawks Professional Football team. He's been a powerful source of inspiration for me. In fact, I even have a pair of Seahawk running shorts that I wear frequently. (I'm pretty sure I run a lot faster when I have them on!) I've adapted his mantra to *"Why not me?"* and employ it whenever I'm overwhelmed with feelings of uncertainty related to my business goals.

Another applicable and well-known mantra is Nike's highly motivational *"Just Do It"* slogan. It's catchy and easy to remember.

I've used it as a powerful source of inspiration when I discover myself stalling and not taking action on something I'm not in the *"mood"* to do or know will be difficult and will push me beyond my comfort zone. I often follow it up by asking myself *"What's the worst that could happen?"*

Finding Your Motivational Mantra

A personal mantra is a *positive affirmation or phrase* that you repeat frequently to yourself for the purpose of encouragement, motivation, strength and/or focusing your mind to achieve your goals.

Reciting a personally motivating mantra, one that resonates with you and your fitness goals, will put you in the right mindset to hang in there when things are tough and to keep moving forward when you want to give up. To be the most effective, mantras need to be repeated frequently. Repetition allows the mantra's meaning to enter into your subconscious and turn your negative thought patterns and habits into beneficial ones.

You'll struggle with different things, and, the things you're struggling with will change depending on what else is happening in your life at that time. Knowing this, it makes sense that creating different mantras for different situations is the most effective way to integrate them into your *cognitive toolbox.*

Motivational mantras can be adapted to "fit" whatever your needs are at any particular time. *Consider your inner motivations and choose a mantra to fit your current needs.* Personal motivational mantras work best if they're short, easy to remember, and sum up what's meaningful to you.

Examples of Motivational Mantras

"Action Conquers Fear."

"I'm worth every drop of sweat!"

"I WILL reach my goal!"

"Okay, workout, let's do this!"

"Strive for progress, not perfection."

"I'm only one workout away from a good mood."

"Just Do It! Then Do It AGAIN!"

"No pain, no gain."

"Giving up is NOT an option!"

"I can. I will. End of Story."

"Excuses are for those who need them."

"Dig Deep!"

"I am powerful."

"I am my own change."

"I can't finish what I don't start."

"I am the author of my own story."

"Losers discuss why they can't."

"Clear your mind of can't."

"There are no shortcuts."

"Pain is temporary, quitting lasts forever."

"Yesterday is NOT today."

"A moment on the lips, forever on the hips."

"Every journey begins with a single step."

"Nothing hurts me more than doing nothing."

"I deserve to be fit and happy."

"I'm doing this for me."

"I'll never know my limits unless I push myself to them."

"I am RELENTLESS!"

Self-empowering mantras can give you a motivational boost even when you're already feeling positive, but they're especially helpful when your spirits are lagging, you're feeling overwhelmed by life, and/or when situational depression and inertia are looming. Finding motivational mantras that speak to your inner self and placing them where they can be daily motivators provides you with support even when no one else is around.

Think about your fitness goals. Find or create a short, easy to remember mantra that targets your reluctance, fear, exhaustion, or disbelief. Repeat it frequently and train your mind to be your most formidable fitness ally.

Summary:

Putting It All Together

Exercise to get and stay fit, not skinny.
Eat to nourish and fuel your body.
And always, always...ignore the haters, doubters, and unhealthy
thoughts that were once feeding your mind.
Love and appreciate your amazing body and your beautiful self.
Take massive action that will transform your life.
Why?
Because you're worth far more than you realize.

Your mindset is the collection of thoughts and beliefs that shape your thought habits. These habits affect how you think, what you feel, and what you do. Developing a habitual mindset that's growth-oriented and infused with realistic optimism is the best frame of mind to promote goal attainment and success. How you choose to handle the ebb and flow of your motivational level will determine how quickly and how well you complete your fitness goals. Building mastery and confidence in other areas of your life will help you get over obstacles that crop up in the path to reaching your fitness goals. And, finally, all of the above feels easier if you're in a good mood.

To achieve your fitness goals:

- Pay attention to how your thinking affects your emotions, mood and behavior.

- Counter negative, self-defeating and self-limiting thoughts.

- Manage your emotions and your stress level.

- Take steps to enhance your mood.

- Cultivate a growth mindset that's augmented with realistic optimism and a general attitude of realistic confidence.

- Set S.M.A.R.T. goals for each fitness component (body, mind, and emotional). Evaluate for effectiveness and then re-evaluate as you make progress.

- Take action, even if your motivation is lacking – sometimes it takes initial action to generate motivation.

- If you find yourself engaging in self-sabotaging behavior, ask yourself the tough questions about your true motivations. Answer the questions honestly. Only then can you determine if you're on the right track and just need to get over the hump or if you need to rethink what your priorities are.

Now that you have a detailed plan that incorporates all three fitness components (body, mind, and emotional); a confident, realistically optimistic, growth-oriented, obstacle crushing mindset; *and*, you're in a positive, upbeat, energetic mood, take advantage of it. Go forth and conquer that treadmill, that workout routine, that new easy, healthy recipe you found!

YOU'VE GOT THIS!

You may not be there yet, but you're closer than you were yesterday!

Motivational Quotes

Augment your use of Motivational Mantras with Motivational Quotes in your brain "re-training" program. Like mantras, quotes are used for encouragement, inspiration, and powerful reminders of why you started your fitness journey in the first place. Quotes are most effective if they're visible and available to you when you most need a motivational "boost." Put them in locations where you know you'll struggle the most: Fitness room, gym bag, refrigerator door, snack cupboard or pantry, closet door, bathroom, mirror, office, and anywhere else you think would be helpful.

This is the poster quote I have hanging in front of my office desk. It helps me adjust my mindset and attitude in all 3 life fitness areas: physical, mental, and emotional. It also serves me well when I'm struggling with the technical side of my business.

"We either make ourselves miserable, or we make ourselves strong. The amount of work is the same." Carlos Castaneda

Here are more quotes that might inspire, encourage, or focus you:

"I already know what giving up feels like. I want to see what happens when I don't." Anonymous

"It's not a short term diet. It's a long term lifestyle change." Anonymous

"Respect your past, your self, your goals, and your aspirations. They're the building blocks for your future." Stephanie Eissinger

"Inaction breeds doubt and fear. Action breeds confidence and courage." Dale Carnegie

"Giving up your goal because of one setback is like slashing your other 3 tires because you got a flat." Anonymous

"Never allow waiting to become a habit. Live your dreams and take risks. Life is happening now." Anonymous

"Lose the self-defeating thoughts and behaviors...instead, adopt a "can do" attitude." Stephanie Eissinger

"Success is focusing the full power of all you are on what you have a burning desire to achieve." Wilfred A. Peterson

"Live less out of habit and more out of intent." Anonymous

"Bad days make for great workouts." Anonymous

"Every positive change in your life begins with a clear, unequivocal decision that you are going to either do something or stop doing something." Anonymous

"Don't let negativity 'live' in your thoughts...like an unwanted house guest, allow it to be a BRIEF visitor and then send it on its way!" Stephanie Eissinger

"In moments of doubt, close your eyes and imagine yourself a year from now. Then, get back to work." Anonymous

"The path of least resistance just makes the road longer. Sometimes you have to head straight on into the pain to come out the other side." recitethis.com

"I trust that there is a purpose behind my challenges." picturequotes.com

"Instead of shying away from challenges and life's ups and downs, meet them head on with enthusiasm, courage and the determination to live life on your terms." Stephanie Eissinger
"You'll never change your life until you change something you do daily. The secret of your success is found in your daily routine." John C. Maxwell

"Fitness is as much psychological as it is physical, master your mind." Anonymous

"Nothing worth having comes easy." Anonymous

"Do something today that your future self will thank you for." Anonymous

"The more you exercise your inner strength, the more resilient you become." Stephanie Eissinger

Remember, with hard work and dedication, you can turn your dreams into goals and your goals into reality! Thank you for sharing part of your fitness journey with me.

Stephanie E.

*** If you'd like to explore the option of Wellness Coaching to help you achieve your Life Fitness Goals, you can contact the author via email at coach@sagebrushcoaching.com.**

APPENDIX

1 – Sample Food Diary

2 – Thoughts, Feelings, Behavior Log

3 – Feelings List

4 – Sample Exercise/Running Log

5 – Sample Life Fitness Goal Plan

One Day Food Diary

Day & Date:

FOOD	TIME	FEELINGS AFTER EATING	REASONS FOR EATING

Thoughts, Feelings & Behavior Log

Triggering Event	Thoughts	Feelings	Behavior

Feelings List

Happy	Sad	Anxious	Afraid	Angry	Assertive
Pleased	Unhappy	Uneasy	Scared	Irritated	Determined
Positive	Hurt	Tense	Threatened	Frustrated	Daring
Wonderful	Upset	Insecure	Weak	Annoyed	Brave
Elated	Lonely	Inadequate	Nervous	Furious	Eager
Excited	Guilty	Trapped	Suspicious	Enraged	Energetic
Content	Miserable	Ashamed	Shocked	Bitter	Inspired
Upbeat	Bereft	Mixed-Up	Surprised	Resentful	Motivated
Proud	Despairing	Confused	Horrified	Destructive	Relaxed
Glad	Devastated	Discontented	Hysterical	Mad	Relieved
Thrilled	Lost	Foolish	Distrustful	Hostile	Satisfied
Forgiving	Let Down	Discomfort	Paranoid	Jealous	Appreciated
Loving	Depressed	Stressed	Betrayed	Envious	Grateful
Ecstatic	Negative	Apprehensive	Disgusted	Hateful	Creative
Curious	Tearful	Embarrassed	Tired	Critical	Thoughtful
Hopeful	Abandoned	Stupid	Exhausted	Flustered	Playful
Peaceful	Disappointed	Disbelieving	Drained	Cross	Nurturing
Optimistic	Grieving	Worried	Pessimistic	Trapped	Compassionate
Confident	Regretful	Bored	Selfish	Spiteful	Powerful
Joyful	Depressed	Discouraged	Disapproving	Contempt	Respected
Thankful	Worthless	Weak	Obstinate	Hopeless	Valuable
Serene	Inferior	Indifferent	Stubborn	Melancholy	Important
Positive	Rejected	Helpless	Exasperated	Humiliated	Triumphant
Valuable	Apathetic	Submissive	Flat	Dejected	Exhilaration
Cheerful	Negative	Cautious	Remorse	Dread	Enthusiastic

This list is not exhaustive. Fill in the blanks with any other feelings you experience.

Sample Exercise/Running Log

MONTH: DAY	DISTANCE	TIME	COURSE/EXERCISE/ WORKOUT	NOTES:
Monday				
Tuesday				
Wednesday				
Thursday				
Friday				
Saturday				
Sunday				
Week's Total:				
Last weeks ytd total:				
Year to date total:				

- Be sure to put the date below the day.
- Put N/A in the distance section if it isn't a run.
- Put the amount of time worked out in the time section if it's not a run.
- Put the type of exercise engaged in or the type of run or course in column two.
- Put notes on weather and temperature (outside runs), heart rate if monitoring, how it felt, difficulty level, purpose, or any other kind of information that you'd like to track in the notes column.
- You can track the number of miles run for the week and year to date or you can track amount of time spent working out in the week's total and year to date total's sections.
  - Tracking your workouts allows you to monitor your progress, hold yourself accountable, and identify patterns that need to be addressed.

Life Fitness Goal Plan

I want to achieve the long range **LIFE Fitness** goal of:

I will do so by _____.(target date)

This goal meets the following goal setting guidelines:

_____1. It's specific and measurable.
_____2. It's achievable. (skills, abilities, strengths, resources)
_____3. It's realistic. (time constraints, accessibility)
_____4. It's time framed. (target date assigned for completion)
_____5. I belief I can do it. (positive & optimistic mental attitude)
_____6. I want to do it.
_____7. I am motivated for the right reasons.
_____8. It's worth setting – I value it.

I want to achieve this goal because it'll be worthwhile (and of value) or potentially satisfying in the following ways:

Personal strengths or abilities I can use to meet my goals are:

What obstacles to achieving my long-range goal do I anticipate?

**Achievement of a goal can sometimes be blocked by you or by external factors. If the block is coming from you, it may be necessary to set and achieve early short-term goals to develop specific skills or to change your attitudes, feelings and thoughts. If the blocks are coming from other people or institutions, you may need to set your short term goals to reduce, overcome or bypass the blocks. But first it'll be necessary to document the reality of any blocks you might expect. Often the "expecting" of blocks, actually creates them. You need to anticipate goal achievement problems before you finalize setting your goal.

How do I plan to overcome these obstacles? (Be specific. Having a plan to meet anticipated obstacles will build confidence in your ability to deal with them if they come up. Sometimes the best defense is having a prepared offense!)

If _____, then I will _____

_____.

If _____, then I will _____

_____.

If_____, then I will _____

_____.

Goal Chunks (smaller, short goals necessary to make progress toward larger, long-range goals)

Short-term **Body Fitness** Goal (first step to meeting long range Life Fitness goal):

_____

_____

- Objective 1:_____

_____

- Objective 2:_____

_____

- Objective 3:_____

_____

*Objectives are the specific, measurable action steps needed to achieve your goal.

I will do this by _____ (target date).

Does this goal meet the goal setting guidelines?

Result:

Short-term **Mind Fitness** goal (goal chunk) to help me achieve my long range Life Fitness goal:

_____

_____

- Objective 1:_____

_____

- Objective2:_____

_____

- Objective 3:_____

_____

I will do this by _____ (target date).

Does this goal meet the goal setting guidelines?

Result:

Short-term **Emotional Fitness** Goal (step to meeting long range Life Fitness goal):

_____

_____

- Objective 1:_____

_____

- Objective 2:_____

_____

- Objective 3: _____

_____

I will do this by _____ (target date).

Does this goal meet the goal setting guidelines?

Result:

Other goals I will need to set to achieve my long range Life Fitness Goal:

Goal:

Objective 1:

Objective 2:

Objective 3:

Date to be Achieved:

Results:

Goal:

Objective 1:

Objective 2:

Objective 3:

Date to be Achieved:

Results:

Goal:

Objective 1:

Objective 2:

Objective 3:

Date to be Achieved:

Results:

I achieved my long range Life Fitness Goal on:

Feelings and thoughts I have about achieving my goal and doing short and long range goal setting are:

How I intend to CELEBRATE my goal success:

If I didn't achieve my goal, what factors were involved?

Is the goal still open for achievement?

Do I want to continue to work at achieving it?

What I will do differently:

Signature:_____Date_____

Additional Self Help Books by This Author

Journey To Self Empowerment: Increase Self Esteem & Self Confidence

The empowering ideas and suggestions will help you take active control of your life, bolster your self esteem and increase your self confidence. You'll learn how to stay empowered within relationships, set and enforce healthy boundaries, embrace being alone, change your mindset, and develop the inner strength you already have.

Stress Management: 40 Tips For De-Cluttering Your "Inner Closet"

Resource of 40 effective strategies to help you manage your acute and chronic stress. Use them to clear your mind of self-defeating thoughts and beliefs, calm your intense emotions, and relieve the tension in your body. Make room inside your "inner closet" for creative thinking, positive thoughts and feelings, and new, empowering beliefs.

Divorce Recovery: How To Clean Out Your "Inner Closet

An essential guide to finding your way to a healthy Divorce recovery and a healthier, happier, more successful future. Grieve your Divorce related losses and find closure, rediscover who you are, and open yourself up to a new chapter in your life.

Upcoming Self Help Books by Stephanie Eissinger:

How To "Rock" Your Body Image: Improve Body Image & Body Confidence

Essential guide to recognizing body image issues, developing a healthier body image, dealing with "fat" days, redefining beauty, building body confidence, and becoming the best version of you. Plus, be inspired by the personal essays of real women with real bodies who have learned to "rock" their body image.

How to Get an "Emotional Divorce" & Speed Up Your Relationship Recovery

A step by step guide on how to detach from toxic emotions that are keeping you chained to a relationship that's no longer viable. Find out how to break free from the past, embrace your "single" status and focus on moving beyond your pain to start building the foundation of a fabulous new future!

**All titles available on Amazon.com.

About the Author

Stephanie Eissinger, MA, LCPC, CPC, is a Licensed Clinical Professional Counselor and a Certified Professional Coach who's professional focus has been on empowering individuals to recover from life's challenges and lead happier, healthier lives. She has both personal and professional experience dealing with the challenges related to disordered eating, body image issues, divorce/relationship recovery, grief, stress management, and excessive exercising. She has a small Coaching practice but is currently devoting most of her time to her writing in order to serve a greater number of people...no matter where they might reside.